NAVIGATING THE LOW IODINE DIET FOR THYROID HEALING:

Mastering the Low Iodine Diet for Wellness

Adams .U. Morris

TABLE OF CONTENTS

CHAPTER 1

Understanding Iodine and Thyroid Health

In our quest to navigate the complexities of a low iodine diet, it's crucial to start at the very beginning: understanding iodine and its pivotal role in thyroid health. The thyroid gland, a small but mighty butterfly-shaped organ nestled in your neck, wields an astonishing degree of influence over your body's overall well-being. To grasp the necessity of a low iodine diet, we must first comprehend the intimate connection between iodine and the thyroid.

The Thyroid Gland: The Body's Metabolic Control Center

Think of your thyroid as the conductor of your body's metabolic orchestra. It orchestrates the tempo at which your cells work, influencing your heart rate, body temperature, and energy production. This tiny powerhouse achieves this control primarily through the secretion of hormones, primarily thyroxine (T4) and triiodothyronine (T3).

These hormones act like messengers, delivering orders to every cell in your body, telling them how fast or slow to perform their specific functions. For instance, if your thyroid is functioning optimally, it ensures your cells metabolize nutrients efficiently, maintaining a stable weight and keeping you energetic. But when things go awry, the consequences can be profound.

Iodine: The Thyroid's Essential Building Block

Now, enter iodine into the scene. Iodine is an essential trace element, which means that your body requires it in minute amounts, yet it's absolutely critical for the proper functioning of your thyroid gland. In fact, it's a key ingredient in the production of thyroid hormones, T4 and T3.

Here's how it works: your thyroid gland is like a factory, and iodine is one of its primary raw materials. The gland takes iodine from your bloodstream and combines it with an amino acid called tyrosine to create T4 (thyroxine), which is named after its four iodine atoms. Some of this T4 is then converted into the more active hormone T3 (triiodothyronine) by removing one iodine atom.

These thyroid hormones are what provide the marching orders to your cells, telling them to either speed up or slow down. If your body doesn't receive enough iodine, it can't produce enough T4 and T3, which leads to a condition known as hypothyroidism, characterized by an underactive thyroid. This, in turn, results in a slowdown of bodily processes, leading to symptoms such as fatigue, weight gain, and cold intolerance.

The Iodine Paradox: Essential Yet Potentially Harmful

Iodine's role as a thyroid essential is undeniable, but there's a paradox here. While you absolutely need iodine, too much of it can be just as problematic as too little.

In areas where iodine deficiency is common, public health initiatives have led to the fortification of salt with iodine, which has successfully eliminated many cases of severe iodine deficiency. However, this fortification can lead to excessive iodine intake when coupled with a diet rich in iodine-containing foods.

Excess iodine can trigger hyperthyroidism, where the thyroid gland becomes overactive. Symptoms can include rapid heartbeat, anxiety, and unintended weight loss. Furthermore, in individuals predisposed to certain autoimmune thyroid diseases like Hashimoto's thyroiditis or Graves' disease, excess iodine can exacerbate the condition.

The Low Iodine Diet Necessity: A Radioactive Twist

So, if we need iodine but not too much of it, why would anyone need to go on a low iodine diet? The answer lies in the management of thyroid disorders and a specific medical procedure: radioactive iodine treatment.

Radioactive iodine therapy is a common approach to treat hyperthyroidism and certain types of thyroid cancer. The idea is to use radioactive iodine, which is selectively absorbed by the thyroid gland, to destroy overactive thyroid cells or cancerous ones. To maximize the therapy's effectiveness, it's crucial to ensure that the thyroid gland takes up as much of the radioactive iodine as possible.

And here comes the catch: if your body is saturated with iodine from your diet, the thyroid may not absorb enough of the radioactive iodine for the treatment to work properly. That's where the low iodine diet comes in. By severely restricting iodine intake for a period before the treatment, it "starves" the thyroid of iodine, making it more receptive to the radioactive iodine.

This dietary strategy plays a crucial role in ensuring the success of radioactive iodine therapy, particularly in cases of thyroid cancer where eliminating all thyroid tissue is often the goal.

Other Instances Where a Low Iodine Diet May Be Prescribed

While radioactive iodine treatment is the most common reason for embarking on a low iodine diet, there are other situations where it might be recommended:

1. **Thyroid Surgery Preparation:** Before thyroid surgery, especially if it involves removing all or

part of the thyroid gland, a low iodine diet may be prescribed. This helps reduce the gland's size and vascularity, making the surgical procedure safer and more manageable.

2. **Thyroid Function Testing:** In some cases, doctors may put patients on a temporary low iodine diet when they suspect thyroid dysfunction but want to assess the gland's natural ability to absorb iodine.

3. **Pregnancy and Lactation:** Pregnant and breastfeeding women have

slightly higher iodine requirements due to the demands of their growing baby. However, excessive iodine intake during this time can also be problematic. In such cases, healthcare providers may provide specific dietary guidance to ensure a balance.

Conclusion of Chapter 1: The Iodine-Thyroid Connection

In Chapter 1, we've delved deep into the intricate relationship between iodine and thyroid health. You've learned how the thyroid gland acts as your body's metabolic conductor and how iodine serves as its essential building block. However, this critical element also presents a paradox; too little or too much iodine can lead to thyroid dysfunction.

Understanding the significance of iodine in thyroid function is the first step toward grasping why a low iodine diet might be necessary. It's a balancing act – ensuring you have enough iodine for a healthy thyroid while avoiding an excess that could lead to problems. In the chapters that follow, we'll explore how to prepare for and navigate the low iodine diet successfully, providing you with the knowledge and tools to maintain optimal thyroid health.

CHAPTER 2

Preparing for the Low Iodine Diet

In Chapter 1, we embarked on a journey to understand the crucial connection between iodine and thyroid health. Now, as we move into Chapter 2, we'll explore the vital steps you need to take before starting a low iodine diet. Preparation is key to success, and it involves not only clearing your pantry of high-iodine foods but also understanding the dietary changes you'll need to make and planning for this unique culinary adventure.

1. Acknowledging the Need for a Low Iodine Diet

Before you even begin preparing for the low iodine diet, it's essential to understand why you need it in the first place. As we discussed in Chapter 1, there are several reasons someone might be prescribed a low iodine diet. It's most commonly associated with preparations for radioactive iodine therapy, but it's also used in specific medical procedures and to manage thyroid conditions.

Understanding the medical necessity of the diet is crucial because it provides motivation and helps you take it seriously. Compliance with the diet's restrictions can significantly impact the effectiveness of your medical treatment or your thyroid health in general.

2. Consultation with a Healthcare Provider

Before embarking on a low iodine diet, it's wise to consult with your healthcare provider. They can provide essential guidance tailored to your specific situation. This consultation should encompass:

- Confirmation of the need for the diet based on your medical condition or procedure.

- Recommendations on the duration of the diet. In most cases, it's short-term, spanning a few days to a couple of weeks.

- Advice on any specific dietary restrictions or considerations due to your health status.

- Discussion of potential side effects, particularly if you have a thyroid condition, and how to manage them during the diet.

Your healthcare provider will be an invaluable source of information and support throughout your journey with the low iodine diet.

3. Clearing Your Pantry and Kitchen

Now, let's dive into the practical aspects of preparing for the low iodine diet, starting with your kitchen. To ensure a smooth transition, it's crucial to remove high-iodine foods from your pantry and refrigerator. These include:

- Iodized salt: Swap it for non-iodized salt or salt substitutes (if your healthcare provider approves).

- Seafood: Any form of seafood, including fish, shellfish, and seaweed, should be eliminated.

- Dairy products: Milk, cheese, and yogurt are typically high in iodine. Replace them with dairy alternatives like almond milk or soy-based products.

- Processed foods: Many processed and pre-packaged foods contain iodized salt and additives rich in iodine. Check labels carefully.

- Some grains and bread: Commercial bread and baked goods often contain iodate dough conditioners. Opt for homemade or bakery bread without these additives.

- Some vegetables: While most vegetables are low in iodine, it's wise to avoid high-iodine options like spinach, kale, and potatoes.

Clearing your kitchen of these items is an essential first step because it eliminates temptation and ensures you're not accidentally consuming high-iodine foods during the diet.

4. Creating a Low Iodine Shopping List

With your kitchen now free of high-iodine culprits, it's time to build a shopping list of low iodine alternatives. The key to success with the diet is knowing what you can eat, not just what you need to avoid. Here's a list of foods to include in your low iodine shopping list:

- Fresh fruits and vegetables: Most fruits and vegetables

are naturally low in iodine. Opt for a variety to ensure you get a range of nutrients.

- Fresh meats: Unprocessed meats like chicken, turkey, pork, and beef are generally safe. Just be sure they're not injected with iodine-containing solutions.

- Eggs: Eggs are a great source of protein and can be incorporated into many low iodine recipes.

- Grains: Rice, pasta, and oats are staples that can form the base of many low iodine meals.

- Non-iodized salt: Stock up on non-iodized salt for seasoning your dishes.

- Fresh herbs and spices: These add flavor without adding iodine.

- Cooking oils: Most cooking oils, like olive oil and vegetable oil, are low in iodine.

Creating a detailed shopping list can help streamline your grocery trips and reduce the chances of accidentally purchasing high-iodine items.

5. Meal Planning and Preparation

A low iodine diet can seem challenging, but with thoughtful meal planning and preparation, it becomes much more manageable. Consider these meal planning tips:

- Breakfast: Opt for oatmeal with fresh fruit or dairy-free yogurt. Eggs and toast are also excellent choices.

- Lunch: Make salads with fresh vegetables, grilled chicken, and a homemade vinaigrette dressing. Rice and beans with sautéed vegetables are another nutritious option.

- Dinner: Grill or bake fresh meats like chicken or turkey and serve them with a side of steamed or roasted low-iodine vegetables.
- Snacks: Keep a supply of fresh fruits, cut-up vegetables, and unsalted nuts on hand for quick and healthy snacks.

Batch cooking can be your best friend during this time. Prepare large quantities of low iodine meals and freeze them in portions. This way, you always have a compliant meal ready when you're short on time or energy.

6.   Educating   Yourself   on Iodine Content

As you delve deeper into your low iodine diet journey, it's helpful to educate yourself about the iodine content of various foods. While many foods are naturally low in iodine, some may surprise you. For example, iodine can be found in unexpected places like some medications and supplements. Learning to read labels and identify potential sources of iodine will help you make informed choices throughout the diet.

7. Emotional Preparation

Lastly, it's essential to prepare yourself emotionally for the low iodine diet. Changing your diet can be challenging, and you may encounter moments of frustration, temptation, or even sadness. However, remember why you're doing this – for your health. Visualize the positive outcomes, stay connected with your support network, and remind yourself that this is a temporary phase.

Conclusion of Chapter 2: Preparing for Success

In Chapter 2, we've walked through the critical steps of preparing for a low iodine diet. It's not just about what you can't eat; it's about understanding the why, consulting with your healthcare provider, clearing your kitchen of high-iodine foods, and stocking up on low iodine alternatives.

Effective preparation is the foundation of a successful low iodine diet. By following these steps, you'll be well-equipped to embark on this journey with confidence, setting the stage for a healthier thyroid and successful medical treatment if needed. In the chapters that follow, we'll delve deeper into the intricacies of the diet, exploring the foods you can enjoy and strategies for navigating social situations and dining out while adhering to these dietary restrictions.

CHAPTER 3

The Basics of a Low Iodine Diet

Having prepared yourself both mentally and practically in Chapter 2, it's time to dive headfirst into the heart of the matter in Chapter 3: understanding the fundamentals of a low iodine diet. In this chapter, we'll explore in detail what you should and shouldn't eat during this dietary journey, providing you with the knowledge needed to confidently navigate your food choices.

1. Foods to Avoid: The Iodine-Rich Offenders

At the core of a low iodine diet is the need to eliminate or significantly reduce your intake of iodine-rich foods. This list primarily includes:

- **Iodized Salt:** This is a big one. It's commonly used in most kitchens, but during your low iodine diet, you should replace it with non-iodized salt. You can find non-iodized salt in most grocery stores, usually labeled as "kosher salt" or "sea salt."

- **Seafood:** Fish, shellfish, and seaweed are among the highest iodine-containing foods. These should be strictly avoided during your diet. Even small amounts can significantly impact your iodine intake.

- **Dairy Products:** Milk, cheese, yogurt, and other dairy products are known to contain iodine, primarily due to the iodine-rich diet of dairy cows. Dairy alternatives like almond or soy milk are better options.

- **Processed and Cured Meats:** Bacon, ham, sausages, and processed deli meats can have added iodine-containing preservatives. Opt for fresh, unprocessed meats instead.

- **Processed Foods:** Many packaged and processed foods contain iodized salt and iodine-containing additives. This includes items like canned soups, frozen dinners, and snacks. Always check the labels for hidden iodine sources.

- **Eggs from Iodine-Fed Hens:** Some commercial egg-laying hens are fed iodine supplements, which can lead to iodine-contaminated eggs. If possible, source your eggs from hens that aren't on iodine-rich diets.

2. Foods to Include: Building a Low Iodine Diet

Now that you know what to avoid let's explore what you can eat:

- **Fresh Fruits and Vegetables:** Most fruits and vegetables are low in iodine and should form the foundation of your low iodine diet. These are rich in essential nutrients, vitamins, and fiber. Some exceptions include high-iodine vegetables like spinach and kale, so it's a good idea to consume them in moderation.

- **Fresh Meats:** Unprocessed meats like chicken, turkey, pork, and beef are generally safe for a low iodine diet. Just be cautious about meats that may have been injected with iodine-containing solutions. Always check labels or ask your butcher for clarification.

- **Eggs:** Eggs, when not sourced from iodine-fed hens, are a valuable source of protein and nutrients during your low iodine diet.

- **Grains:** Rice, pasta, and oats are excellent staples for a low iodine diet. They're versatile and can be used in a variety of dishes.

- **Non-Iodized Salt:** As mentioned earlier, non-iodized salt is your go-to seasoning during this diet. Use it for flavoring your meals and recipes.

- **Fresh Herbs and Spices:** These are your secret weapons for adding flavor to your dishes without adding iodine. Experiment with herbs like basil, oregano, thyme, and spices like garlic and onion powder.

- **Cooking Oils:** Most cooking oils, such as olive oil, vegetable oil, and canola oil, are low in iodine and can be used for cooking and dressing your salads.

3. Hidden Iodine Sources: Reading Labels Carefully

Navigating a low iodine diet also means becoming a label detective. Hidden sources of iodine can sometimes lurk in unexpected places, even in products you wouldn't suspect. Here are some potential hidden sources to be aware of:

- **Medications and Supplements:** Certain medications and supplements can contain iodine. Always consult your healthcare provider about any potential iodine content in your medications.

- **Iodine-Based Sanitizers:** Some sanitizers and disinfectants used in food processing can leave trace amounts of iodine on the surface of fruits, vegetables, or even kitchen equipment. A thorough rinse and cleaning can help reduce this risk.

- **Restaurant and Fast Food:** Dining out can be a challenge during a low iodine diet. Many restaurant dishes are prepared with iodized salt or iodine-containing ingredients. It's best to communicate your dietary restrictions to the restaurant staff and inquire about menu options that can be tailored to your needs.

- **Vitamins and Minerals:** Some multivitamins and mineral supplements may contain iodine. Double-check the labels or consult with a healthcare provider for suitable alternatives.

4. Managing Sodium Intake

Sodium is a critical component of salt, and during a low iodine diet, you'll be relying on non-iodized salt for seasoning. However, it's essential to be mindful of your overall sodium intake. Excessive sodium can lead to high blood pressure and other health issues.

To manage your sodium intake:

- Use non-iodized salt sparingly. A little goes a long way in adding flavor to your meals.
- Embrace fresh herbs, spices, and other flavorings like lemon juice or vinegar to enhance the taste of your dishes without relying solely on salt.
- Be cautious with processed meats, as they can be high in

sodium, even if they don't contain iodine.

5. Monitoring Your Iodine Intake

As you navigate your low iodine diet, it's essential to keep track of your iodine intake. This can be particularly crucial if you're preparing for a medical procedure like radioactive iodine therapy. To monitor your iodine intake:

- Keep a food diary: Write down everything you eat and drink, including portion sizes.

- Use online resources and iodine content charts: Several online databases provide information on the iodine content of various foods.

- Consult with your healthcare provider or a registered dietitian: They can offer guidance on managing your iodine intake and may even recommend iodine testing to ensure you're on track.

Conclusion of Chapter 3: Navigating the Low Iodine Diet

In Chapter 3, we've delved deep into the basics of a low iodine diet, providing you with a comprehensive understanding of what to include and exclude from your meals. Armed with this knowledge, you're now well-equipped to embark on your low iodine dietary journey.

Remember, while the restrictions may seem daunting, this is a temporary phase with significant benefits for your thyroid health or medical treatment. In the chapters that follow, we'll explore practical strategies for preparing delicious low iodine meals, managing social situations, and maintaining motivation throughout your journey.

CHAPTER 4

Delicious Low Iodine Recipes

Now that you've grasped the fundamentals of a low iodine diet, it's time to embark on a culinary adventure in Chapter 4. This chapter is dedicated to introducing you to a collection of flavorful and iodine-free recipes that will not only make your low iodine diet more enjoyable but also showcase the variety of delicious meals you can still savor while adhering to your dietary restrictions.

1. Breakfast Delights

Recipe 1: Oatmeal with Fresh Berries

- Ingredients:
    - 1 cup of rolled oats
    - 2 cups of water
    - 1 cup of fresh berries (blueberries, strawberries, or raspberries)
    - 1 tablespoon of honey (optional)
    - A pinch of non-iodized salt

Instructions:

1. Bring water to a boil in a saucepan.

2. Add oats and a pinch of salt. Reduce heat and simmer for about 5 minutes, stirring occasionally until the oats are tender.

3. Remove from heat and let it sit for a minute. Serve topped with fresh berries and a drizzle of honey if desired.

Recipe 2: Scrambled Eggs with Herbs

- Ingredients:
  - 2 large eggs

- o 1 tablespoon of chopped fresh herbs (e.g., parsley, chives, or basil)
- o A pinch of non-iodized salt
- o 1 tablespoon of olive oil

Instructions:

1. Crack the eggs into a bowl and beat them lightly with a fork.
2. Heat olive oil in a non-stick skillet over medium-low heat.

3. Pour the beaten eggs into the skillet and stir gently as they cook.

4. Add chopped herbs and a pinch of non-iodized salt while stirring.

5. Cook until the eggs are set but still slightly moist. Serve immediately.

2. Lunchtime Bliss

Recipe 3: Grilled Chicken and Vegetable Salad

- Ingredients:
  - 2 boneless, skinless chicken breasts

- 2 cups of mixed fresh vegetables (e.g., bell peppers, zucchini, and cherry tomatoes)
- 2 tablespoons of olive oil
- Juice of one lemon
- Fresh herbs (e.g., basil or oregano) for seasoning
- A pinch of non-iodized salt

Instructions:

1. Preheat your grill to medium-high heat.
2. Brush the chicken breasts and vegetables with olive oil.

3. Season the chicken with fresh herbs and a pinch of non-iodized salt.

4. Grill the chicken for about 6-7 minutes per side until it's cooked through, and the vegetables until they're tender and slightly charred.

5. Slice the chicken and serve it over a bed of grilled vegetables. Drizzle with fresh lemon juice.

Recipe 4: Lentil and Vegetable Soup

- Ingredients:
    - 1 cup of dried green or brown lentils

- o 4 cups of vegetable broth (ensure it's low in iodine)
- o 2 cups of diced mixed vegetables (carrots, celery, and onions)
- o 2 cloves of garlic, minced
- o 1 tablespoon of olive oil
- o Fresh herbs (e.g., thyme or rosemary) for seasoning
- o A pinch of non-iodized salt

Instructions:

1. Heat olive oil in a large pot
    over medium heat. Add
    minced garlic and sauté until
    fragrant.
2. Add diced vegetables and
    cook for about 5 minutes
    until they begin to soften.
3. Add lentils, vegetable broth,
    fresh herbs, and a pinch of
    non-iodized salt.
4. Bring the soup to a boil, then
    reduce the heat to low,
    cover, and simmer for 25-30
    minutes until the lentils are
    tender.
5. Serve hot and garnish with
    additional fresh herbs if
    desired.

3. Satisfying Dinners

Recipe 5: Baked Salmon with Lemon and Herbs (For Non-Radioactive Iodine Diet)

- Ingredients:
    - 2 salmon fillets
    - Juice of one lemon
    - 1 tablespoon of olive oil
    - Fresh herbs (e.g., dill or parsley) for seasoning
    - A pinch of non-iodized salt

Instructions:

1. Preheat your oven to 375°F (190°C).

2. Place salmon fillets on a baking sheet lined with parchment paper.

3. Drizzle with olive oil and lemon juice.

4. Season with fresh herbs and a pinch of non-iodized salt.

5. Bake for about 15-20 minutes until the salmon flakes easily with a fork. Serve hot.

Recipe 6: Spaghetti Aglio e Olio (Garlic and Olive Oil Pasta)

- Ingredients:

- 8 oz (225g) of spaghetti
- 3 cloves of garlic, thinly sliced
- 3 tablespoons of olive oil
- Red pepper flakes (optional)
- Fresh parsley for garnish
- A pinch of non-iodized salt

Instructions:

1. Cook spaghetti according to package instructions until al dente. Drain and set aside.

2. Heat olive oil in a skillet over medium heat. Add sliced garlic and red pepper flakes (if using). Cook until the garlic turns golden.

3. Add cooked spaghetti to the skillet and toss to coat with the garlic-infused olive oil.

4. Season with a pinch of non-iodized salt and garnish with fresh parsley. Serve hot.

4. Snacktime Treats

Recipe 7: Homemade Trail Mix

- Ingredients:

- o 1 cup of unsalted nuts (e.g., almonds, cashews, or walnuts)
- o 1 cup of dried fruit (e.g., raisins, apricots, or cranberries)
- o 1 cup of unsalted sunflower seeds
- o 1 cup of unsalted pumpkin seeds
- o A pinch of non-iodized salt

Instructions:

1. Mix all the ingredients in a large bowl.

2. Store in an airtight container for a convenient, iodine-free snack.

Recipe 8: Fruit Kabobs

- Ingredients:
    - A selection of fresh fruit (e.g., pineapple, strawberries, and melon)
    - Wooden skewers

Instructions:

1. Wash and cut the fruit into bite-sized pieces.
2. Thread the fruit onto wooden skewers to create colorful and tasty kabobs.

Conclusion of Chapter 4: Exploring Delicious Low Iodine Recipes

In Chapter 4, we've embarked on a culinary journey to discover delicious low iodine recipes that can make your dietary restrictions not only manageable but enjoyable. These recipes showcase the versatility of a low iodine diet, proving that you can still savor a wide range of flavors and dishes while prioritizing your thyroid health or medical treatment.

By incorporating these recipes into your meal planning, you'll not only maintain your compliance with the low iodine diet but also embrace a palate of tastes that might surprise you. In the chapters that follow, we'll delve into practical strategies for managing social situations, dining out, and staying motivated on your low iodine diet journey.

CHAPTER 5

Dining Out and Social Situations

Navigating a low iodine diet isn't just about what you eat at home. It extends to how you handle dining out and social situations. In Chapter 5, we'll explore practical strategies to help you maintain your dietary restrictions while still enjoying restaurant meals and social gatherings.

1. Communicating Your Dietary Needs

One of the first and most crucial steps when dining out is to effectively communicate your dietary needs. Whether you're dining at a restaurant or attending a social event, don't hesitate to let others know about your low iodine diet. Here's how you can do it:

- **At Restaurants:**
    - Call ahead: If possible, call the restaurant in advance to discuss your dietary restrictions with the staff. This can help ensure they are prepared to

accommodate your needs.

- o Speak to the server: When you arrive at the restaurant, inform your server about your dietary requirements. They can guide you through the menu and check with the kitchen to accommodate your needs.
- o Ask questions: Don't hesitate to ask questions about how dishes are prepared and what ingredients are used. For example,

inquire about the type of salt they use for seasoning.

- **At Social Gatherings:**
  - Notify the host: If you're attending a social event at someone's home, reach out to the host ahead of time to explain your dietary restrictions. They may be willing to prepare a dish or offer alternatives.
  - Offer to bring a dish: To ensure you have something safe to eat, offer to bring a low

iodine dish to share with others. This way, you can enjoy the meal without worrying about your dietary restrictions.

2. Choosing Safe Menu Items

When dining out, selecting the right menu items can make all the difference. Here are some guidelines for choosing safe options:

- **Opt for Plain Preparations:** Look for dishes that are prepared simply, without sauces, seasonings, or toppings that may contain iodized salt or iodine-rich ingredients.

- **Ask for Customization:** Don't be afraid to ask for modifications to suit your dietary needs. For example, request grilled chicken without seasoning or sauces.

- **Stick to Fresh Ingredients:** Choose dishes that feature fresh, whole ingredients like vegetables, fruits, and unprocessed proteins.

- **Beware of Hidden Iodine:** Be cautious about items that may contain hidden iodine, such as sushi, which often contains seaweed and iodine-rich seafood.

3. Dining Out Strategies

Dining out can be enjoyable even on a low iodine diet if you approach it strategically:

- **Research Ahead of Time:** Before choosing a restaurant, research their menu online. Many restaurants provide detailed menus on their websites, which can help you identify safe options in advance.

- **Call in Advance:** If you have specific questions or concerns about the menu, call the restaurant ahead of time to discuss your dietary restrictions.

- **Plan Your Orders:** Have an idea of what you'll order before you arrive at the restaurant. This can help you avoid feeling overwhelmed when making choices on the spot.

- **Pack Your Own Seasoning:** Consider carrying a small container of non-iodized salt with you when dining out. This way, you can season your dishes to your liking.

- **Bring Snacks:** In case your dining options are limited, keep a few low iodine snacks in your bag to tide you over until you can enjoy a full meal.

4.   Navigating   Social Situations

Social gatherings, from parties to family dinners, can present unique challenges on a low iodine diet. Here's how to navigate these situations gracefully:

- **Communicate in Advance:** If you're attending a social event where food will be served, inform the host about your dietary restrictions well in advance. This gives them time to plan accordingly.

- **Offer to Contribute:** Consider offering to bring a low iodine dish to the event. This not only ensures you have a safe option to eat but also allows you to share your dietary journey with others.

- **Eat Beforehand:** If the menu at a social event isn't conducive to your dietary needs, eat a small meal or snack beforehand so you're not ravenous when you arrive.

- **Be Polite and Grateful:** When declining food offerings or explaining your dietary restrictions, be polite and appreciative. Most people are understanding and willing to accommodate.

- **Educate When Appropriate:** If someone asks about your diet, use it as an opportunity to educate them about thyroid health and the importance of a low iodine diet in certain medical situations.

5. Staying Motivated

Maintaining motivation on a low iodine diet can be challenging, especially when faced with tempting high-iodine foods in social settings. Here are some strategies to stay motivated:

- **Focus on Your Health:** Remind yourself why you're following this diet. Whether it's for thyroid health or medical treatment, keeping your health as the primary goal can help you stay committed.

- **Set Realistic Expectations:** Understand that there may be moments of frustration or temptation. Acknowledge these feelings, but don't let them deter you from your goal.

- **Plan Rewards:** Consider setting up small rewards for yourself as milestones. For example, treat yourself to a special non-food item or activity when you successfully complete a week on the diet.

- **Lean on Support:** Share your journey with friends and family who can offer encouragement and understanding. Joining a support group or seeking guidance from a registered dietitian can also be immensely helpful.

- **Get Creative:** Experiment with new recipes and cooking techniques to keep your meals interesting and satisfying.

6. Handling Dining Out Challenges

Despite your best efforts, dining out challenges may still arise. Here's how to handle them:

- **Mistakes Happen:** If you accidentally consume something that violates your dietary restrictions, don't be too hard on yourself. Mistakes can happen, and they don't erase your overall progress.

- **Take Precautions:** If you suspect a mistake or cross-contamination at a restaurant, be cautious about any potential side effects, and contact your healthcare provider if you experience any unusual symptoms.

- **Learn and Adapt:** Use any challenges or mistakes as opportunities to learn and adapt. Consider what led to the issue and how you can prevent it in the future.

Conclusion of Chapter 5: Dining Out and Social Situations

In Chapter 5, we've explored practical strategies for dining out and navigating social situations while adhering to a low iodine diet. Effective communication, menu selection, planning, and staying motivated are key components of successfully maintaining your dietary restrictions in various scenarios.

Remember that a low iodine diet is a temporary journey with important benefits for your thyroid health or medical treatment. By following the guidance in this chapter, you can confidently enjoy meals at restaurants, attend social events, and stay on track with your diet, all while prioritizing your well-being. In the chapters that follow, we'll delve deeper into monitoring your progress, managing challenges, and maintaining your thyroid health in the long term.

CHAPTER 6

Monitoring Progress and Long-Term Thyroid Health

As you've journeyed through the previous chapters of this guide, you've gained a deep understanding of the low iodine diet, from its necessity for thyroid health to practical strategies for preparing delicious meals, dining out, and navigating social situations. Now, in Chapter 6, we shift our focus to monitoring your progress during the diet and the importance of long-term thyroid health.

1. Monitoring Your Iodine Intake

Throughout your low iodine diet, it's essential to monitor your iodine intake. This monitoring serves multiple purposes:

- **Compliance:** It ensures that you're adhering to the dietary restrictions as prescribed by your healthcare provider. Staying compliant is crucial for the effectiveness of medical treatments or the management of thyroid conditions.

- **Adjustment:** Regular monitoring allows you to make adjustments if necessary. If you find that your iodine intake is higher than desired, you can take steps to correct it, such as modifying your food choices or portion sizes.

Here's how you can monitor your iodine intake:

- **Food Diary:** Continue to keep a detailed food diary. Write down everything you eat and drink, including portion sizes. This diary provides a clear picture of your daily iodine consumption.

- **Use Iodine Content Charts:** Utilize iodine content charts and databases, which are available online or through medical resources. These resources can help you estimate the iodine content of various foods.

- **Consult with Healthcare Providers:** Regularly consult with your healthcare provider or a registered dietitian who can provide guidance on monitoring and adjusting your iodine intake as needed.

2. Managing Challenges and Setbacks

As with any dietary journey, challenges and setbacks may arise during your low iodine diet. It's essential to approach these situations with resilience and problem-solving skills:

- **Unexpected Iodine Sources:** Despite your best efforts, you may encounter unexpected iodine sources. For instance, certain medications or supplements may contain iodine. If you suspect any such sources, discuss them with your healthcare provider.

- **Dining Out Mishaps:** Mistakes or cross-contamination can happen when dining out. If you suspect you've consumed iodine by accident, don't panic. Instead, focus on learning from the experience and preventing it in the future.

- **Social Gatherings:** Social events can pose challenges, as not everyone may be aware of your dietary restrictions. Remember the strategies discussed in Chapter 5 to navigate these situations gracefully.

- **Coping with Frustration:** Staying motivated throughout the diet can be challenging, especially when faced with tempting high-iodine foods. When frustration sets in, remind yourself of your health goals, seek support from loved ones, and consider rewards for your progress.

3. Post-Diet Evaluation and Thyroid Health

Once you've successfully completed your low iodine diet, it's important to evaluate the impact of the diet on your thyroid health and overall well-being. Here's what this evaluation entails:

- **Medical Assessments:** Schedule follow-up appointments with your healthcare provider to assess your thyroid health. This may involve blood tests, imaging studies, or other diagnostic tools to determine the effectiveness of the diet or the status of your thyroid condition.

- **Review of Progress:** During these appointments, discuss your dietary journey with your healthcare provider. Share your food diary and any challenges you faced. This information can guide future treatment decisions.

- **Long-Term Thyroid Health:** Even after completing the low iodine diet, maintaining long-term thyroid health is essential. Continue to work closely with your healthcare provider to manage any thyroid conditions, take prescribed medications, and follow recommended treatment plans.

- **Thyroid Health Education:** Educate yourself about thyroid health and thyroid conditions. Understanding your condition and treatment options empowers you to make informed decisions and advocate for your well-being.

4. Transitioning to a Balanced Diet

After completing the low iodine diet and receiving guidance from your healthcare provider, it's time to transition back to a balanced diet that supports your thyroid health. Here are some steps to facilitate this transition:

- **Gradual Reintroduction:** Reintroduce high-iodine foods gradually to avoid overwhelming your system. Start by adding small portions of iodine-containing foods back into your diet.
- **Continue Monitoring:** Maintain a watchful eye on

your iodine intake, especially if you have a thyroid condition. Periodically monitor your progress, ideally with guidance from a registered dietitian.

- **Thyroid-Boosting Foods:** Incorporate foods that are beneficial for thyroid health into your regular diet. These include selenium-rich foods like Brazil nuts, zinc-rich foods like beans, and omega-3 fatty acids found in fatty fish like salmon.

- **Balanced Nutrition:** Focus on a well-balanced diet that includes a variety of nutrient-rich foods. This promotes overall health and supports your thyroid's optimal function.

- **Stay Hydrated:** Proper hydration is essential for thyroid health. Ensure you're drinking an adequate amount of water daily.

- **Regular Exercise:** Engage in regular physical activity, as it can help manage thyroid conditions and promote overall well-being.

5. Maintaining Motivation for Long-Term Health

Maintaining motivation for long-term thyroid health is a journey in itself. Here are some strategies to keep you motivated:

- **Set Goals:** Establish clear and achievable health goals related to your thyroid condition. Having concrete objectives can give you a sense of purpose.

- **Seek Support:** Lean on your support network, whether it's friends, family, or support groups for individuals with thyroid conditions. Share your experiences, concerns, and triumphs.

- **Stay Informed:** Stay up-to-date with developments in thyroid health, treatment options, and dietary recommendations. Knowledge empowers you to make informed choices.

- **Celebrate Progress:** Celebrate your successes, no matter how small they may seem. Each step forward is a testament to your dedication to your health.

- **Mind-Body Practices:** Consider incorporating mind-body practices like yoga, meditation, or deep breathing exercises into your routine. These can help manage stress and promote a sense of calm.

6. The Role of a Registered Dietitian

Throughout your journey of monitoring progress and maintaining long-term thyroid health, a registered dietitian can be an invaluable resource. They can:

- **Provide Guidance:** A dietitian can offer expert advice on maintaining a balanced diet that supports your thyroid health.

- **Create Personalized Plans:** They can develop personalized meal plans that meet your specific dietary needs and restrictions, taking into account your thyroid condition.

- **Monitor Progress:** A dietitian can help you monitor your iodine intake, assess your nutritional status, and make adjustments as necessary.

- **Offer Education:** Dietitians can educate you about the connection between nutrition, thyroid health, and overall well-being.

- **Address Concerns:** If you have any concerns or questions about your diet or thyroid health, a dietitian is there to provide answers and support.

Conclusion of Chapter 6: Monitoring Progress and Long-Term Thyroid Health

In Chapter 6, we've explored the importance of monitoring your progress during and after the low iodine diet and the significance of maintaining long-term thyroid health. Completing the diet is just one step in your thyroid health journey. Regular medical assessments, a balanced diet, a supportive network, and informed choices are all essential components of your ongoing commitment to your well-being.

Remember that your health is a lifelong journey, and it's perfectly normal to face challenges along the way. With dedication, knowledge, and support, you can effectively manage your thyroid health and enjoy a fulfilling life. Continue to work closely with your healthcare provider and consider the guidance of a registered dietitian to ensure that your thyroid health remains a top priority.

CHAPTER 7

Thyroid Health and Lifestyle

In this final chapter, we'll delve into the intricate relationship between your thyroid health and lifestyle factors. Your thyroid gland plays a pivotal role in regulating various bodily functions, and several aspects of your lifestyle can impact its function. We'll explore these connections and provide practical guidance on how to maintain a thyroid-friendly lifestyle.

1. The Thyroid's Crucial Role

Before delving into the impact of lifestyle on thyroid health, let's briefly revisit the essential role the thyroid gland plays in your body:

- **Metabolism Regulation:** Your thyroid gland produces thyroid hormones, primarily thyroxine (T4) and triiodothyronine (T3). These hormones play a crucial role in regulating your metabolism, which affects how your body uses energy and manages weight.

- **Energy Production:** Thyroid hormones influence

how efficiently your body produces and uses energy. An imbalance in thyroid hormones can lead to fatigue or excess energy.

- **Temperature Control:** Thyroid hormones help regulate your body temperature. An underactive thyroid can lead to feeling cold, while an overactive thyroid can cause excessive heat.

- **Heart and Digestive Function:** Your thyroid affects heart rate and digestive processes. Imbalances can lead to irregular heartbeats or digestive issues.

- **Brain and Nervous System:** Thyroid hormones influence brain development, mood, and cognitive function. Thyroid disorders can affect mental health and cognitive performance.

Now, let's explore lifestyle factors that can impact thyroid health:

2. Nutrition and Thyroid Health

Proper nutrition is fundamental for maintaining a healthy thyroid.

Here's how diet can influence your thyroid:

- **Iodine:** As discussed throughout this guide, iodine is essential for thyroid hormone production. A diet either excessively high or low in iodine can disrupt thyroid function. For individuals with thyroid conditions, maintaining an appropriate iodine intake is crucial.
- **Selenium:** Selenium is a mineral that plays a role in converting T4 to the more active T3 hormone.

Incorporating selenium-rich foods like Brazil nuts, whole grains, and lean meats into your diet can support thyroid health.

- **Tyrosine:** Tyrosine is an amino acid necessary for thyroid hormone production. Foods like lean protein, dairy products, and nuts contain tyrosine and can contribute to thyroid function.

- **Cruciferous Vegetables:** Some cruciferous vegetables, such as broccoli, cabbage, and Brussels sprouts, contain compounds that can interfere with thyroid function when consumed in large amounts. Cooking these vegetables can help reduce their impact.

- **Gluten and Dairy:** Some individuals with thyroid conditions, particularly Hashimoto's thyroiditis, may benefit from reducing or eliminating gluten and dairy from their diets. These foods can sometimes trigger autoimmune responses.

- **Balanced Nutrition:** Overall, maintaining a well-balanced diet rich in fruits, vegetables, lean proteins, whole grains, and healthy fats supports thyroid health and overall well-being.

3. Exercise and Thyroid Health

Regular physical activity is another lifestyle factor that can positively impact thyroid health:

- **Weight Management:** Exercise can help with weight management, which is crucial for individuals with thyroid conditions. Weight fluctuations can affect thyroid function.

- **Metabolism Boost:** Physical activity can boost metabolism, helping your body efficiently use energy. This can be especially beneficial for those with an underactive thyroid (hypothyroidism).
- **Stress Reduction:** Exercise is an effective stress reducer. Chronic stress can contribute to thyroid dysfunction, so finding healthy ways to manage stress is important.
- **Improved Mood:** Exercise releases endorphins, which can improve mood and

alleviate symptoms of depression or anxiety that are sometimes associated with thyroid conditions.

- **Bone Health:** Some thyroid disorders, especially hyperthyroidism, can affect bone health. Weight-bearing exercises can help maintain bone density.

- **Balanced Approach:** While exercise is generally beneficial, individuals with thyroid conditions should listen to their bodies and avoid overtraining, which can lead to fatigue.

4. Stress Management and Thyroid Health

Chronic stress can negatively impact thyroid health in several ways:

- **Hormone Imbalance:** Prolonged stress can disrupt hormone balance, including thyroid hormones. This can exacerbate existing thyroid conditions.

- **Immune Function:** Stress weakens the immune system, making individuals more susceptible to autoimmune thyroid disorders like Hashimoto's or Graves' disease.

- **Thyroiditis Triggers:** Stress can trigger thyroiditis, an inflammation of the thyroid gland. This can lead to temporary thyroid dysfunction.

- **Medication Effectiveness:** Stress can affect how the body metabolizes thyroid medications, potentially altering their effectiveness.

Effective stress management is crucial for thyroid health. Strategies include:

- **Relaxation Techniques:** Practice relaxation techniques such as deep breathing, meditation, or progressive muscle relaxation to reduce stress.

- **Regular Exercise:** As mentioned earlier, regular physical activity can be a powerful stress reliever.

- **Sleep:** Prioritize good sleep hygiene to ensure you're getting enough rest. Lack of sleep can exacerbate stress.

- **Support Systems:** Lean on friends, family, or support groups to share your experiences and receive emotional support.

- **Professional Help:** Consider seeking help from a therapist or counselor if you're struggling to manage stress on your own.

5. Sleep and Thyroid Health

Quality sleep is essential for overall health, and it plays a role in thyroid function as well:

- **Hormone Regulation:** Sleep is a critical time for hormone regulation, including thyroid hormones. Consistent, restorative sleep supports healthy hormone levels.

- **Energy Levels:** A lack of sleep can lead to fatigue and reduced energy levels, which can exacerbate symptoms of thyroid conditions like hypothyroidism.

- **Immune Function:** Sleep is essential for a well-functioning immune system. Adequate rest can help prevent or manage autoimmune thyroid disorders.

To promote better sleep:

- **Establish a Routine:** Go to bed and wake up at the same time each day to regulate your body's internal clock.

- **Create a Relaxing Bedtime Ritual:** Wind down before bed with calming activities such as reading, stretching, or taking a warm bath.

- **Limit Stimulants:** Avoid caffeine and electronics before bedtime, as they can interfere with sleep.

- **Comfortable Sleep Environment:** Ensure your bedroom is conducive to sleep with a comfortable mattress, dark curtains, and a comfortable room temperature.

- **Physical Activity:** Regular exercise can improve sleep quality, but avoid vigorous activity close to bedtime.

6. Medications and Thyroid Health

For many individuals with thyroid conditions, medications are a critical component of managing their health:

- **Hypothyroidism Medications:** Individuals

with an underactive thyroid (hypothyroidism) typically require synthetic thyroid hormone replacement medications, such as levothyroxine. It's essential to take these medications as prescribed to maintain proper thyroid hormone levels.

- **Hyperthyroidism Medications:** For hyperthyroidism, treatment may involve medications to reduce thyroid hormone production or block its effects. Adherence to medication regimens is crucial.

- **Thyroid Function Monitoring:** Regularly monitoring thyroid function through blood tests is essential to ensure medication effectiveness and appropriate dosages.

- **Interaction Awareness:** Be aware of medications or supplements that can interact with thyroid medications. Discuss any new medications or supplements with your healthcare provider.

7. Thyroid Health and Smoking

Smoking can have detrimental effects on thyroid health:

- **Increased Risk:** Smoking is associated with an increased risk of developing thyroid disorders, particularly Graves' disease.
- **Thyroid Antibodies:** Smoking can lead to increased levels of thyroid antibodies, which are markers of autoimmune thyroid diseases like Hashimoto's thyroiditis.

- **Medication Interference:** Smoking can interfere with the effectiveness of thyroid medications.

If you smoke, quitting is one of the best steps you can take to support your thyroid health and overall well-being. Seek support from healthcare professionals or smoking cessation programs to quit successfully.

8. Alcohol and Thyroid Health

Moderation is key when it comes to alcohol and thyroid health:

- **Liver Function:** Excessive alcohol consumption can harm liver function, which plays a role in converting thyroid hormones. This can disrupt thyroid function.

- **Medication Interactions:** Alcohol can interact with thyroid medications, affecting their absorption and metabolism.

- **Hypothyroidism Risk:** Some studies suggest a link between alcohol consumption and an increased risk of hypothyroidism.

If you choose to consume alcohol, do so in moderation, and discuss your alcohol consumption with your healthcare provider to ensure it aligns with your thyroid treatment plan.

9. Environmental Factors and Thyroid Health

Environmental factors, such as exposure to certain chemicals and pollutants, can impact thyroid health:

- **Endocrine Disruptors:** Some chemicals found in pesticides, plastics, and household products can disrupt thyroid function by interfering with hormone production and regulation.

- **Radiation Exposure:** Excessive exposure to radiation, whether from medical treatments or environmental sources, can damage the thyroid gland and lead to thyroid disorders.

- **Iodine Exposure:** In regions with high iodine intake, excessive exposure to iodine can lead to thyroid dysfunction.

To minimize environmental risks:

- **Limit Exposure:** Be mindful of exposure to potentially harmful chemicals, especially in cleaning products and plastics.

- **Radiation Safety:** Follow safety guidelines for medical procedures involving radiation. If you work in an environment with radiation exposure, take appropriate precautions.

- **Monitor Iodine Intake:** If you live in an area with high iodine levels in the water or diet, consult with your healthcare provider to ensure your iodine intake is within the recommended range.

10. Regular Thyroid Check-Ups

Regardless of your lifestyle choices, regular check-ups with your healthcare provider are paramount for maintaining thyroid health:

- **Thyroid Function Tests:** These tests, including TSH (thyroid-stimulating hormone), T4, and T3, help monitor thyroid function and hormone levels.

- **Physical Examination:** A physical examination may reveal thyroid nodules or enlargement.

- **Ultrasound:** If necessary, your healthcare provider may recommend an ultrasound to assess the thyroid gland's structure and look for abnormalities.

- **Thyroid Antibody Tests:** For autoimmune thyroid disorders like Hashimoto's or Graves' disease, antibody tests can provide valuable diagnostic information.

- **Medication Adjustment:** Based on test results, your

healthcare provider can make necessary adjustments to your thyroid medications to maintain optimal hormone levels.

11. Thyroid Health and Aging

Thyroid function can change with age:

- **Hypothyroidism:** Older individuals are more likely to develop hypothyroidism. Regular thyroid check-ups become increasingly important as you age.

- **Osteoporosis Risk:** Aging and thyroid dysfunction can

both contribute to bone loss (osteoporosis). Adequate calcium and vitamin D intake and weight-bearing exercise are crucial.

- **Medication Adjustments:** As you age, your thyroid medication needs may change. Regular monitoring helps ensure appropriate dosage.

12. Patient Advocacy and Education

Ultimately, you are your best advocate for thyroid health:

- **Educate Yourself:** Continue to educate yourself about thyroid health, your specific thyroid condition, and treatment options.

- **Ask Questions:** Don't hesitate to ask your healthcare provider questions and seek clarification about your diagnosis, treatment plan, and lifestyle recommendations.

- **Seek Second Opinions:** If you have concerns or doubts about your diagnosis or treatment, seeking a second opinion can provide valuable insights.

- **Participate in Decisions:** Be an active participant in your healthcare decisions. Collaborate with your healthcare team to make informed choices.

Conclusion of Chapter 7: Thyroid Health and Lifestyle

In Chapter 7, we've explored the intricate interplay between your thyroid health and various lifestyle factors, from nutrition and exercise to stress management and environmental considerations. Your thyroid gland, a master regulator of metabolism and vital bodily functions, is influenced by the choices you make in your daily life.

By prioritizing a balanced diet, regular exercise, stress management, and adherence to prescribed medications, you can support your thyroid health and overall well-being. Remember that thyroid conditions may require ongoing monitoring and adjustment of your lifestyle choices to ensure optimal health outcomes. Be proactive in advocating for your thyroid health, seek support from healthcare professionals, and stay informed to make the best decisions for your unique journey to thyroid wellness.

CHAPTER 8

Thyroid Health for Life

Congratulations on reaching the final chapter of this comprehensive guide to thyroid health! In Chapter 8, we will explore the concept of long-term thyroid health and provide you with valuable insights on how to maintain optimal thyroid function throughout your life. While previous chapters focused on the low iodine diet, dining out, lifestyle factors, and more, this chapter will help you consolidate your knowledge and take proactive steps to ensure that your thyroid remains healthy for the long haul.

1. The Ongoing Journey

First and foremost, it's important to understand that managing thyroid health is a lifelong journey. Whether you have a thyroid condition or simply want to maintain optimal thyroid function, consistency in your approach is key. The strategies discussed in this chapter will help you navigate this journey effectively.

2. Regular Check-Ups and Monitoring

Regular check-ups and monitoring of your thyroid function are critical elements of maintaining long-term thyroid health. Here's what you need to know:

- **Frequency of Check-Ups:** The frequency of thyroid check-ups will depend on your specific thyroid condition and your healthcare provider's recommendations. Generally, individuals with thyroid disorders should undergo annual thyroid function tests.

- **Thyroid Function Tests:** These tests include TSH (thyroid-stimulating hormone), T4, and T3 measurements. They provide valuable insights into your thyroid hormone levels and overall thyroid function.

- **Physical Examination:** During check-ups, your healthcare provider may perform a physical examination to check for thyroid nodules, enlargement, or other abnormalities.

- **Ultrasound and Imaging:** If deemed

necessary, your provider may recommend an ultrasound or other imaging tests to assess the thyroid gland's structure.

- **Antibody Tests:** For autoimmune thyroid disorders like Hashimoto's or Graves' disease, antibody tests can be conducted to monitor disease activity.

- **Medication Adjustments:** Based on test results, your healthcare provider may make adjustments to your thyroid medications to ensure you maintain optimal hormone levels.

3. Medication Adherence

If you're taking thyroid medications, adherence to your prescribed regimen is crucial for maintaining thyroid health. Here's how to ensure medication adherence:

- **Set a Routine:** Take your medication at the same time each day to establish a routine. Consider incorporating it into a daily habit, such as brushing your teeth.

- **Medication Alerts:** Use medication reminder apps or alarms on your phone to prompt you when it's time to take your medication.

- **Refill Prescriptions Early:** Ensure you never run out of medication by refilling your prescription a few days before it's due to run out.

- **Storage:** Store your medication as directed, typically at room temperature and away from moisture and direct sunlight.

- **Communicate with Your Provider:** If you experience

side effects or any issues related to your medication, communicate with your healthcare provider. They can adjust your prescription if needed.

4. Dietary Considerations

Diet plays a significant role in supporting long-term thyroid health. Consider the following dietary tips:

- **Iodine Monitoring:** If you've been following a low iodine diet due to a thyroid condition, continue monitoring your iodine intake. Work with a registered dietitian to ensure you strike the right balance between adequate iodine and avoiding excess.

- **Balanced Nutrition:** Maintain a well-balanced diet rich in fruits, vegetables, lean proteins, whole grains, and healthy fats. This provides essential nutrients for overall health, including thyroid function.

- **Selenium-Rich Foods:** Include selenium-rich foods like Brazil nuts, whole grains, and lean meats in your diet, as selenium supports thyroid health.

- **Tyrosine Sources:** Consume foods rich in tyrosine, an amino acid necessary for thyroid hormone production. These include lean protein, dairy products, and nuts.

- **Limit Cruciferous Vegetables:** While cruciferous vegetables offer numerous health benefits, if you have thyroid concerns, consider cooking them to reduce their potential impact on thyroid function.

- **Stay Hydrated:** Proper hydration supports all bodily functions, including thyroid health. Ensure you're drinking an adequate amount of water daily.

5. Weight Management

Maintaining a healthy weight is essential for thyroid health. Here's why it matters:

- **Hypothyroidism and Weight Gain:** Individuals with an underactive thyroid (hypothyroidism) often experience weight gain or difficulty losing weight.

Managing weight is crucial for symptom control and overall well-being.

- **Hyperthyroidism and Weight Loss:** Conversely, hyperthyroidism can lead to unintentional weight loss. In such cases, maintaining a healthy weight is about preventing excessive weight loss.

- **Metabolism Support:** A balanced diet and regular exercise are key components of managing your weight and supporting metabolism.

- **Consult with a Healthcare Provider:** If

you're struggling with weight management in relation to your thyroid condition, consult with your healthcare provider or a registered dietitian. They can provide tailored guidance and support.

6. Stress Management

Chronic stress can negatively impact thyroid health. Here are strategies for effective stress management:

- **Stress Reduction Techniques:** Incorporate relaxation techniques into your daily routine, such as deep breathing, meditation, or yoga.

- **Physical Activity:** Regular exercise is an excellent way to manage stress. Find physical activities you enjoy and make them a part of your routine.

- **Adequate Sleep:** Prioritize good sleep hygiene to ensure you're getting enough rest. Lack of sleep can exacerbate stress.

- **Support Systems:** Lean on friends, family, or support groups to share your experiences and receive emotional support.

- **Professional Help:** If you're struggling to manage stress on your own, consider seeking help from a therapist or counselor.

7. Environmental Awareness

Environmental factors can impact thyroid health. Stay vigilant and take precautions:

- **Chemical Exposure:** Be mindful of exposure to potentially harmful chemicals, especially in cleaning products and plastics. Choose natural cleaning products when possible.

- **Radiation Safety:** Follow safety guidelines for medical procedures involving radiation. If you work in an environment with radiation exposure, take appropriate precautions.

- **Iodine Levels:** If you live in an area with high iodine levels in the water or diet, consult with your healthcare provider to ensure your iodine intake remains within recommended ranges.

8. Support and Advocacy

Advocating for your thyroid health and seeking support when needed are vital aspects of long-term well-being:

- **Stay Informed:** Continue to educate yourself about thyroid health, your specific thyroid condition, and treatment options.

- **Ask Questions:** Don't hesitate to ask your healthcare provider questions and seek clarification about your diagnosis, treatment plan, and lifestyle recommendations.

- **Participate in Decisions:** Be an active participant in your healthcare decisions. Collaborate with your healthcare team to make informed choices.

- **Second Opinions:** If you have concerns or doubts about your diagnosis or treatment, seeking a second opinion can provide valuable insights.

9. Thyroid Health and Aging

As you age, thyroid function can change. Here's what to keep in mind:

- **Increased Risk of Hypothyroidism:** Older individuals are more likely to develop hypothyroidism. Regular thyroid check-ups become increasingly important as you age.
- **Bone Health:** Aging and thyroid dysfunction can both contribute to bone loss (osteoporosis). Adequate calcium and vitamin D intake and weight-bearing exercise are crucial.

- **Medication Adjustments:** As you age, your thyroid medication needs may change. Regular monitoring helps ensure appropriate dosage.

10. Patient Empowerment and Advocacy

Empowerment and advocacy are central to maintaining long-term thyroid health:

- **Education:** Continue to educate yourself about your thyroid condition and stay informed about

developments in thyroid
health.

- **Ask Questions:** Don't be
afraid to ask your healthcare
provider questions and seek
clarification.

- **Participate in Decisions:**
Be actively involved in your
healthcare decisions,
working collaboratively with
your healthcare team.

- **Second Opinions:** If you
have concerns or doubts
about your diagnosis or
treatment, seeking a second
opinion can provide peace of
mind.

Conclusion of Chapter 8: Thyroid Health for Life

In Chapter 8, we've explored the essential concepts and strategies for maintaining optimal thyroid health throughout your life. Your thyroid is a vital gland that impacts numerous bodily functions, and it requires ongoing attention and care.

Regular check-ups, medication adherence, a balanced diet, stress management, environmental awareness, and patient advocacy are all integral components of your long-term thyroid health journey. By prioritizing these aspects, you can enjoy a healthy and fulfilling life, with your thyroid functioning at its best. Remember that you are not alone in this journey; healthcare providers, support networks, and educational resources are available to assist you along the way. Here's to a lifetime of thyroid wellness!

CONCLUSION

In conclusion, this comprehensive guide has taken you on a journey through the intricacies of thyroid health, from understanding the thyroid's role in the body to practical strategies for managing your thyroid health effectively. Let's recap some key takeaways from each chapter:

Chapter 1: The Thyroid Demystified

- The thyroid gland is a small but powerful organ responsible for regulating metabolism and many bodily functions.

- Thyroid conditions can lead to imbalances in hormone production, affecting your overall health.

Chapter 2: Thyroid Disorders Demystified

- Common thyroid disorders include hypothyroidism (underactive thyroid) and hyperthyroidism (overactive thyroid).
- Autoimmune conditions like Hashimoto's and Graves' disease can also affect the thyroid.

Chapter 3: Diagnosing Thyroid Disorders

- Diagnosis of thyroid disorders involves blood tests to measure thyroid hormone levels and other diagnostic tools like ultrasound and radioactive iodine scans.

- Accurate diagnosis is crucial for determining the appropriate treatment.

Chapter 4: Thyroid Treatment Options

- Treatment for thyroid disorders varies depending

on the specific condition but can include medication, radioactive iodine therapy, or surgery.

- Regular monitoring and adjustments are often necessary to maintain thyroid health.

Chapter 5: The Low Iodine Diet

- The low iodine diet is a temporary dietary restriction designed to reduce iodine intake, primarily in preparation for radioactive iodine therapy or thyroid scans.

- It involves avoiding high-iodine foods like iodized salt, seafood, and dairy products.

Chapter 6: Monitoring Progress and Long-Term Thyroid Health

- Monitoring iodine intake is crucial during and after the low iodine diet to ensure compliance and make adjustments as needed.

- Managing challenges, staying motivated, and transitioning back to a balanced diet are essential for long-term thyroid health.

Chapter 7: Thyroid Health and Lifestyle

- Lifestyle factors like nutrition, exercise, stress management, and sleep play significant roles in supporting thyroid health.

- Being aware of environmental factors, medications, and the impact of smoking and alcohol is essential.

Chapter 8: Thyroid Health for Life

- Maintaining long-term thyroid health requires

regular check-ups, medication adherence, a balanced diet, stress management, and environmental awareness.

- Patient empowerment and advocacy are key to making informed decisions about your thyroid health.

In essence, your thyroid health is a lifelong commitment that involves a combination of medical management and personal choices. It's essential to work closely with your healthcare provider, stay informed, and advocate for your well-being.

Remember that you're not alone in this journey; there are resources, support networks, and healthcare professionals available to assist you. By taking proactive steps to manage your thyroid health, you can enjoy a fulfilling and healthy life. Here's to a future filled with thyroid wellness and overall well-being!